a mornir

qigong™

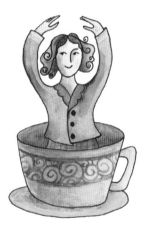

The publisher and author cannot be held responsible for injury, mishap, or damages incurred during the performance of the exercises in this book. The author recommends consultation with a healthcare professional before beginning this or any other exercise program.

"A Morning Cup of" is a trademark of Crane Hill Publishers, Inc.

Published by Crane Hill Publishers
www.cranehill.com

Printed in China

Library of Congress Cataloging-in-Publication Data

Bright-Fey, John A.
   A morning cup of qigong : one 15-minute routine to rebuild your life / by John A. Bright-Fey.
      p. cm.
   ISBN-13: 978-1-57587-244-5
   ISBN-10: 1-57587-244-7
   1. Qi gong. I. Title.
   RA781.8.B75 2006
   613.7'14--dc22

                              2005016607

10   9   8   7   6   5   4   3   2   1

a morning cup of
qigong™

one 15-minute routine to release the natural
energy of your mind and body

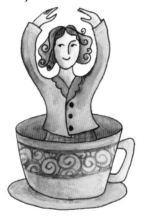

john a. bright-fey

CRANE HILL
PUBLISHERS

Acknowledgments

I'd like to thank the following individuals for their invaluable help and advice. This Morning Cup would surely not taste as sweet without their assistance:

To all of my inspiring and wonderful students around the globe who keep the campfires blazing in the New Forest;

To Ellen, Allison, and all the staff at Crane Hill Publishers for presenting me with this glorious opportunity;

To Charles Fechter, life-long friend and Boswell, for his continuing support during the project;

To Miles Parsons, Tim Rocks, and Christena Brooks for bringing the New Forest to life;

To my amazing wife, Kim, for her boundless love and tireless efforts to bring the wonders of the New Forest to the world;

To all of you, much love and many thanks.

JB-F

This book is lovingly dedicated to the memories of Qigong Masters
Chi and Soo
You stomped the terra
Thank You

Contents

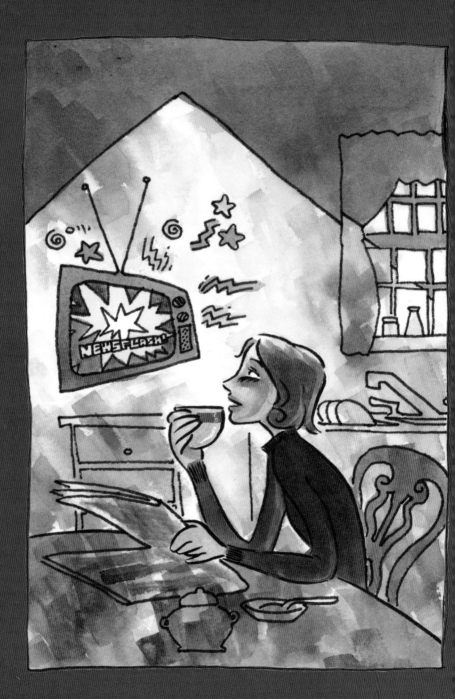

What is Qigong?

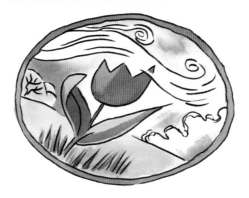

Announcer: "Flash! This just in! What is Qigong? Some people call it Chinese yoga, but it's more than that. It is the most exciting and revolutionary system of whole-body exercise to ever come around. It tones and strengthens the body. It stimulates the mind and reduces stress. It makes you feel vibrant, robust, and full of life. In short, you can look good and feel great!

"Every day, more and more people around the globe are discovering the wonders of Qigong and are beginning to realize that it's nothing short of a modern exercise miracle. No special clothing or exercise equipment is required. These exercises, designed by leading medical scientists, are simple and direct, and the sessions themselves fit easily into anyone's hectic schedule.

"Thoroughly tested under the most rigorous of conditions, these exercises can be done standing up, sitting down, or even while walking around the park. Anyone can do Qigong! Super-athletes become more super. Weekend warriors will use less liniment, and those who have considered themselves to be non-athletic will discover that they, too, can take charge of their fitness needs. Oh! And, by the way, this modern exercise miracle is more than 3,000 years old."

The Wonders of Qigong

In Chinese, Qi means "life-force energy" and gong means "to work" or "to acquire a skill with." It is pronounced "chee-gung." Some people spell it Chi-Kung, but it is pronounced the same way and means the same thing.

Archaeologists tell us that the first book on Qigong was written on bronze and published, as it were, around 1000 BCE in China. By then, the ancient Chinese already knew that Qigong was a modern miracle that promoted great wellness and a zest for living. It wasn't long before it infused nearly every facet of their lives and culture.

Famous philosophers, doctors, and generals practiced Qigong. Science, literature, music, painting, poetry, and even business practices were informed and elevated by the practice of Qigong. In reality, it's almost impossible to talk about any part of ancient Chinese culture without a discussion of Qigong. This is because everything humans do requires energy, and Qigong, as the name implies, is the art of energy — specifically, it is the art of life-energy.

The Simple Secret of Play

Modern life can be very hectic, stressful, and demanding. A busy job or family life consumes a lot of energy and can take a tremendous toll. Modern science tells us that exercise can help manage the stress of everyday living, but all too frequently, a conventional exercise regimen merely adds to the body and mind stresses instead of alleviating them. Sometimes, it can get so overwhelming that it seems as if life runs over us altogether, and no matter how hard we try, we just can't get back on our feet.

During my years as a Qigong and Tai Chi teacher, I've had prospective students ask if there was a way they could be constantly in shape and in tune with the flow of day-to-day living so life couldn't run over them. "Yes," I tell them, "There is. The secret is Qigong."

Qigong is a marvelous and simple way to get the most out of what life has to offer. Anyone can do Qigong, no matter what your physical gifts or deficits. Qigong helps you feel better and look great. It clears your head, lifts your spirits, and helps you live life to the fullest. It puts you in touch with your intuitive and creative side. Qigong fortifies your strengths and diminishes your weaknesses. It reduces stress, promotes healing, and gives you a calm edge over a turbulent world. And all you have to do to reap this bounty is to play for 15 minutes a day: that's right, I said play. In the time it would take for you to have a pleasant cup of tea or coffee, you can harmonize your talent, vision, body, mind, and spirit into a unified whole. Then, instead of life getting smaller, darker, and depressing, it gets bigger, brighter, funnier, and more rewarding by the minute. Couldn't we all stand to play like that?

During the more than forty years I've been playing Qigong on a daily basis, it has never ceased to amaze me. When I'm lacking in basic human gumption, it props me up. If I can't find the answer to a problem, it cuts back the mental confusion so I can see a solution. Wherever I go and whomever I meet, Qigong shows me how to connect not only with the outside world, but with my inside world as well. Playing Qigong has introduced me to great knowledge, power, beauty, wellness, and love. Since I was a teenager, I've referred to Qigong as "romancing my soul." Now, with this Morning Cup, you can romance yours as well.

John A. Bright-Fey
Birmingham, Alabama
Spring 2006

Getting Started

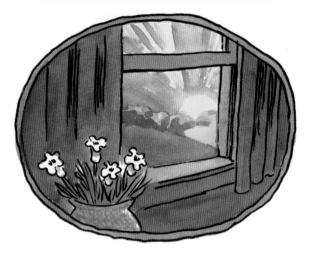

Most people think that learning Qigong is a complicated affair, but that simply isn't true. It is no more complicated than playing a child's game and no more mysterious than a smile. The style and approach to Qigong we will use for our Morning Cup is the New Forest® style. This is my signature approach to the art that puts the many benefits and wonders of Qigong immediately at your fingertips. More importantly, New Forest Qigong is easy to learn and fun to do. I've taught this Qigong to my students for more than twenty-five years, and the result has been nothing short of miraculous.

The next two sections are a concise introduction to Qigong and its basic principles. The routine begins on page 33 and is a presentation of 10 simple Qigong exercises. The extra sips that follow the routine contain more detailed information about your new art, information that I trust will be both useful and interesting. I will show you how to artistically weave Qigong into your daily life so its magic will be with you always.

The last sip is a presentation of my Aphorisms of New Forest Qigong. These ten games will supercharge your Qigong. They represent the distilled wisdom and advice of more than twelve generations of Qigong masters and practitioners. Much of this wisdom has long been regarded as secret and was reserved for only the most dedicated of students. I learned these secrets from many wonderful and generous men and women whose goal was to help me have a more complete and enlightening experience of life. Now, I get to do the same thing for you.

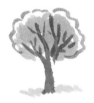

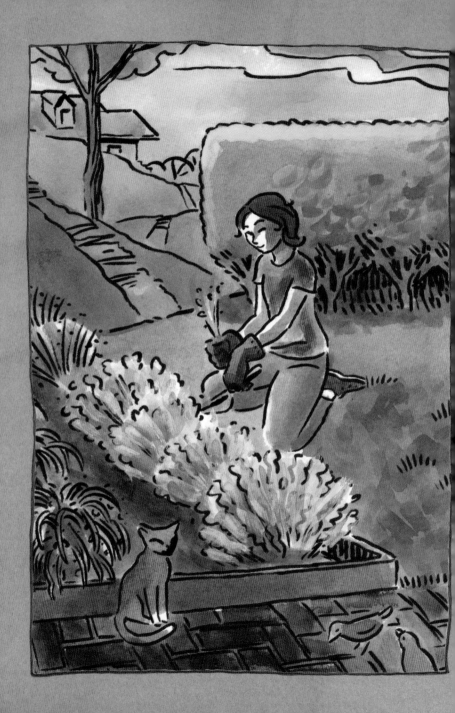

How Qigong Works

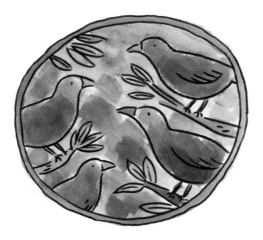

Qigong is a bodymind exercise that creates robust wellness and health by cultivating the Qi, or life-force energy. I use the word bodymind because Qigong players (as they like to be called) will coordinate a specific physical activity with a specific mental one. These two activities form a dynamic inner game that harnesses the life-force energy, generating a profound effect on the whole human organism. If this sounds scientific to you — and it should — it's because extensive field research has been conducted in real-life environments for thousands of years.

During ancient times, Qigong players painstakingly experimented and researched to find just the right physical and mental activities that best go together to generate abundant life-force energy and wellness. Along the way, they discovered the secrets of breath control and meditation, infusing both into their art. As their sensitivity and awareness of Qi increased, they made other discoveries as well: acupuncture, herbology, and massage. In fact, the whole science of Traditional Chinese Medicine is based on Qigong principles. Modern by ancient Chinese standards, the slow-motion dance of Tai Chi is a style of Qigong. The art of placement and landscaping known as Feng-shui was created by Qigong players. Understanding the ways Qi moves across the land and through houses has its roots in the knowledge of how the life-force energy moves through the bodymind. There were other discoveries as well: the compass, gunpowder, the fundamental principles of flight, and even complex mathematical formulae were invented by Qigong players seeking a deeper understanding of their inner and outer worlds. As the first organized natural scientists, Qigong players sought to penetrate the force and mystery of life by cultivating the life-force: the mysterious Qi.

It's All About the Qi

Everything has Qi (life-force energy), including you. Even rocks and cars and air have Qi. But because you are a living being, you have lots more of it. An abundance of Qi in your bodymind signifies a robust life, while deficient Qi levels indicate problems. These problems can be emotional, physical, or even intellectual, because your bodymind needs Qi to do anything from thinking about painting the garage to actually getting around to painting it.

We get a certain amount of Qi from our mothers at birth. Thereafter, we absorb Qi from our environment, the air we breathe, and the food we eat. New Forest Qigong is carefully constructed to help us absorb ever-increasing levels of Qi from our environment and the air we breathe. Furthermore, it moves and distributes this Qi evenly throughout our bodyminds so that our whole organism can benefit. It even excites the Qi we already have to higher levels, and we end up bristling with life-force energy.

Popular books on the subject subdivide Qi into different types, such as pre-birth Qi, post-birth Qi, and ancestral Qi, but these distinctions are not important for now. All you really need to know at this point is that playing Qigong (1) helps you absorb fresh Qi from your surroundings and the air you breathe, (2) distributes the fresh Qi evenly inside of you, and (3) excites your Qi to a high level, enlivening your body, your mind, and your spirit.

Ching-Lo: Energy Pathways

The Qi in your bodymind moves along a specific series of pathways called Ching-Lo, or meridians. These meridians are energy pathways that link up and cross-connect all of your organs, bones, and tissues into one coordinated holistic unit. The best way to understand Ching-Lo theory is to think of them as a series of roads and bridges that form an intricate superhighway system. This system — complete with access roads, overpasses, underpasses, rest stops, and weigh stations — is so finely constructed that Qi in your left pinky toe can travel to your right little finger. If you think about your bodymind's life-force as the cars and trucks that traverse these roads, then your understanding of Ching-Lo theory is almost complete.

When the traffic on your superhighway system is evenly distributed and flowing smoothly, you are in a state of ease. But if one of your bridges is being repaired or if there is an accident that is blocking traffic on a stretch of road, then a state of dis-ease exists.

The soft flowing movements of Qigong, coordinated with breath and imagination repair damaged roads and bridges, clear away accidents and congestion, while directing your inner flow of Qi to go merrily on its way. The acupuncturist uses needles and massage to do exactly the same thing, but that's what's so great about Qigong — you can do it yourself.

It's really very simple: if you feel like this ...

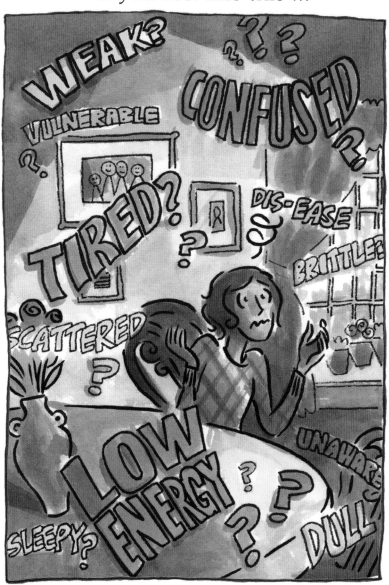

then play New Forest Qigong, and
you'll begin to feel like this ...

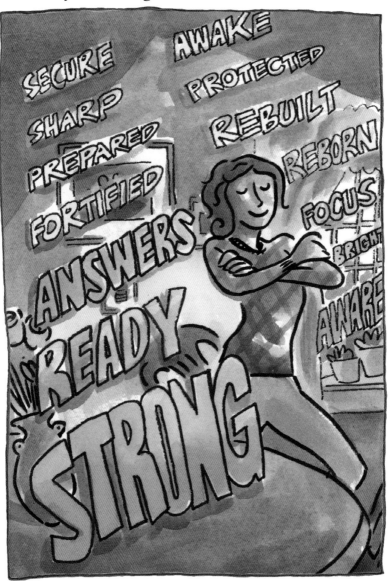

New Forest Qigong

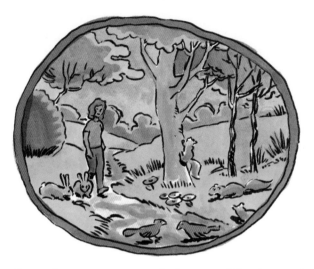

New Forest Qigong is composed of ten carefully chosen physical movements. Each of these movements, which are performed slowly and deliberately, has a just-as-carefully-chosen mental activity or visualization that goes with it. I call these visualizations "internal adjustments" because they alter and adjust the way you inwardly relate to the specific physical Qigong movements. When each of the ten physical movements and visualizations are balanced with one another, the Qi begins to flow smoothly through you. Then you automatically move from a place of less life-force energy to abundant life-force energy — from less Qi to more Qi.

New Forest Qigong is designed to be done either standing up or sitting down. Obviously, you'll get more benefits when standing, but it's your choice. Personally, I like to alternate. One day I'll play my Qigong standing and the next sitting in a chair or cross-legged on cushions.

Learning the physical movements of New Forest Qigong is straightforward enough. I'll explain this in detail as we move through the exercises. Feel free to adjust the postures and movements so they are comfortable for you to do. What's so great about New Forest Qigong is that you can change and adapt the exercises without diminishing their effectiveness. This is not true of other styles of Qigong. I designed New Forest Qigong to be purposefully open and flexible to accommodate the greatest range of body types and the widest variety of personalities. Our modern culture of exercise has unfortunately evolved into a "feel the burn" mentality; that is, if exercise doesn't hurt, then you aren't exercising. This is nonsense. Any new exercise can be physically difficult at first, but you deserve comfort, so make your Qigong movements as big or as small as you would like. Remember, the best exercise in the world for you is the exercise that's fun for you to do and that you will do regularly.

Qigong Breath

Many Qigong and Tai Chi teachers love Chinese calligraphy. I'm no exception. The flowing lines created by brush and ink remind us of our Qigong movements. One of the basic tenets of Chinese brushwriting centers around the coordination of breath with the act of painting. Essentially, the calligrapher gently inhales as he prepares to write a character and then exhales as the brush is put to paper. The breath then gently guides the brush. Whether you are painting a flower, bug, or a Chinese word, how you breathe is considered to be very important. Not only does it affect the beauty of whatever you paint, it also relaxes your body, clears your mind, and enlivens your senses.

The breath carries a special human signal with it that fixes whatever you are doing in emotional space and time. Said another way, it makes whatever you're doing more real and more authentic. I believe it allows a portion of your soul to express itself in whatever movement you perform. Breath coordinated with motion is so important to Chinese painters and calligraphers that we call it the "Artist's Breath of Life" or the "Poet's Breath." We will use the same kind of breathing when we play our Qigong. It will allow us to get deeply inside each of our Qigong postures so the movements and their internal adjustments can work their magic on our bodyminds.

Qigong breathing is really very easy. Whenever your hands move up doing a Qigong movement, you inhale. Whenever your hands move down doing a Qigong movement, you'll exhale. Whenever your hands come in toward your body, you'll inhale. Whenever they move away from your body, you'll exhale. Whenever you twist your waist, you'll breathe out, and whenever your waist untwists, you'll breathe in.

When playing Qigong, ask yourself to move and breathe slowly, but don't force your breath to be slower than is comfortable. Let the natural speed of your breathing tell you how fast to move. The bodymind has great wisdom if we will only listen to it. For Qigong beginners, it's not necessary to coordinate the breath with the movements, but it is something that you should shoot for as you become more experienced. If coordinating your breathing with your movements is confusing, or if your breathing is impaired in any way, just breathe naturally as you move slowly and deliberately through each of the ten exercises. As you become a more experienced Qigong player, your breathing will naturally relax and deepen on its own. Then you will be able to match your Qigong movements with your breathing.

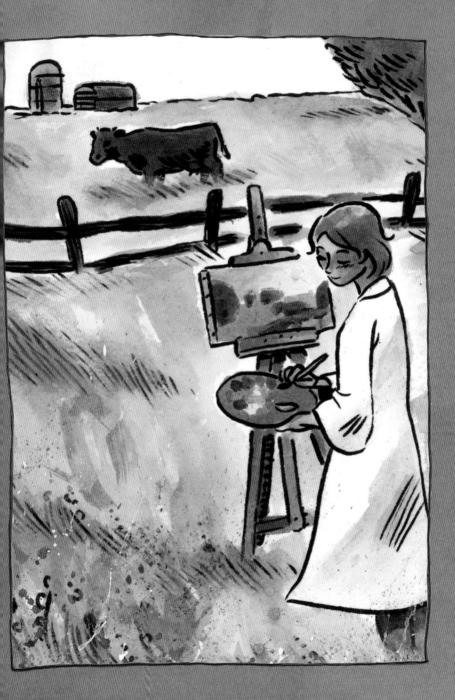

The New Forest "1 through 10" Game

Qigong is sometimes called Nei-gung (pronounced "nay-gong"), which means "esoteric, hidden, or inner work." This is because so much of what gives Qigong its unique strength and character takes place deep inside your bodymind. Simply losing yourself in mindless slow-motion exercise is not the authentic Qigong way. The Qigong movements that you make with your hands and arms must be meaningful if they are to transform you.

I first began using rhyming games and simple number shapes in childhood to help remember how to perform the complex movements of archaic Chinese Qigong. I would twist and bend short poems and nonsense rhymes in my mind so that I'd have a way to translate old Chinese postures and ideas into a form I could easily remember. After all, to an American child, most of the Chinese ideas and movements weren't culturally relevant. They came from Chinese medicine, dance, art, and philosophy. They were not meaningful to me. But the poems, rhymes, and number shapes gave me a basic structure to relate to. Eventually, I could use them to explain any Qigong posture or movement, no matter how detailed or complicated. It allowed me to get deeply inside the Qigong activities.

As I worked to master Chinese art, poetry, movement, and philosophy, I created other mnemonics, including numbering and rhyming games, to help me comprehend their depths. Again, I used numbers to connect the internal secrets and philosophical roots of each exercise to its physicality. I also used these games to bring poetry and music to a physically expressive level. Eventually, I infused Qigong into everything I did!

Now, as a teacher, I use the same memory and number games to help my students. They find that their Qigong is much easier to learn. More importantly, the meaning and the purpose of each Qigong activity becomes almost instantly accessible, just as it did for me decades earlier.

The Qigong movements that we're about to learn are easy and fun to do. You should have no trouble at all picking them up. But if you're to truly get in touch with your inner self, you need to learn the New Forest Qigong "1 Through 10" Game.

If you can count from one to ten, you can play Qigong. It's as easy as that. The New Forest "1 Through 10" keywords will introduce you to the inner landscape of Qigong. Start by reading the following list aloud.

NUMBER	KEYWORD
One	FUN
Two	SHOE
Three	TREE
Four	CORE
Five	ALIVE
Six	THICK
Seven	HEAVEN
Eight	GATE
Nine	SHINE
Ten	SPIN

Now, close your eyes and count from one through ten, saying the numbers and their keywords from memory. Recite silently or aloud, you choose. If you get stuck, open your eyes and read the list again until you know all of the keywords and their associated number. It won't be long before you have them easily memorized. Each keyword tells you what to think about when you play its associated Qigong movement.

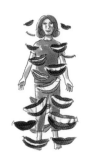

1-FUN

Think of fun. Smile gently and suggest to yourself to relax all over. You can even think of something funny! Enjoy the moment.

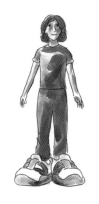

2-SHOE

Think about your toes, feet, and the shoes you're usually wearing standing firmly on the ground. Feel the earth beneath your feet.

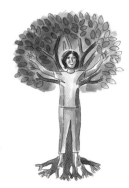

3-TREE

Imagine you are a huge healthy tree with massive branches full of leaves and roots penetrating deeply into the soil. You are rooted, vibrant, and stable.

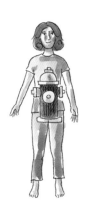

4-CORE

Imagine that you have a fire hydrant buried deep inside your abdomen. This hydrant, located roughly three and a half inches below your navel and inward toward the center of your body, is the place where you gather strength. It is your point of focus.

5-ALIVE

Pretend that pressurized life-giving water from your 4-Core is rushing out of your arms and legs at an incredible rate of speed. It's as if your arms and legs are high-pressure fire hoses and your hands and feet are the nozzles.

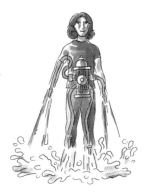

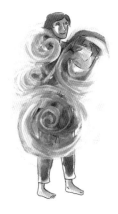

6-THICK

Pretend that all of the air around you is thick and viscous. It's so thick, in fact, you can feel it squishing through your fingers as you move. Imagine that if you relaxed completely, the thick air would cradle you and keep you from falling.

7-HEAVEN

Gently stretch up with the top of your head toward the heavens as if you were a marionette. Pretend you are being lifted subtly upward, rising above the noise and confusion of the moment. Think about something that is important to you: family, friends, religion, your goals, and higher ideals.

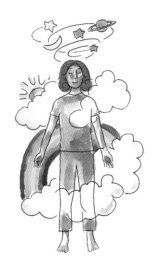

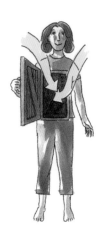

8-GATE

Imagine that each pore of your skin is in reality a tiny gate. As you inhale, these gates swing open and draw air into them, into your bodymind. When you exhale, pretend that the gates close shut and all the life-giving energy from the air around you now circulates freely throughout your entire bodymind.

9-SHINE

Imagine you're a light bulb. That's right: a giant you-shaped light bulb. As you inhale, your light is dim, but you gradually shine out brighter and brighter as you exhale. You are glowing with high-wattage brilliance.

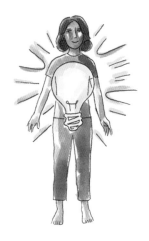

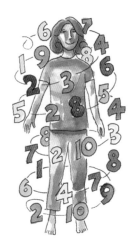

10-SPIN

Let the first nine numbers and their associated images float through your mind in any order. If one pops up in your mind with more clarity than the other, focus on it briefly, and then let it slip away until another comes up. Just let the numbers swirl and spin in your imagination.

The Magic of the Numbers

Although you'll be thinking about the "1 Through 10" internal adjustments when you play your Qigong, you can think about them any time you see a number or a group of numbers. Remember you are using these visualizations to adjust your internal landscape so you can have a greater experience of the outside world. And who among us couldn't stand to be more relaxed (1-Fun) with our feet firmly planted on the ground (2-Shoe); stable, strong, and rooted (3-Tree); more focused (4-Core); more giving (5-Alive); more supported by and connected to our surroundings (6-Thick); more uplifted and inspired (7-Heaven); taking life as it comes to us (8-Gate); pushing back gloomy darkness with a bright sunny disposition (9-Shine) while going with the flow of life (10-Spin)? Get the idea?

Before they became mathematics, numerals themselves were considered to be magical. Indeed, the use of numbers in scientific calculations do effect great change in the modern world around us, but ancient man felt that simply thinking about them in a proper way would cause beneficial change in the outside world. Now, with the "1 Through 10" Game, they can be magical again as you use them to create health and wellness within your inner world.

Qigong gets its astonishing magic and power for health and wellness from the balanced coordination of movement with visualization. That having been said, some days our imagination just doesn't work as well as it does on others. So, does this mean that our Qigong won't work? Of course it will! Each of the physical exercises is designed to move life-force energy in your bodymind in a specific way, whether you are thinking about the appropriate internal adjustment or the mortgage payment. As the physical exercises gradually shape your Qi, you will naturally be led to greater awareness of each of the internal adjustments. In effect, your body will train your mind. It goes the other way, too. Some days, you will feel physically clumsy or not very graceful. Not to worry, though. Focusing on the internal adjustments will begin to shape your Qi until it starts to affect the way you physically move and look. At this point, your mind will be training your body. This is the miracle of Qigong: your mind teaches your body, and your body teaches your mind.

The Importance of Play

While Qigong is an incredible tool for cultivating health and wellness, it has a marvelous multidimensional character that can be applied to almost any human endeavor. It has the power to enhance any life that it meets, that is, any life that is willing to play a little.

Real Qigong people don't often use words like "work out," "train," or "exercise" to describe what they do. They say "play" instead. Lewis Carroll, the Victorian author of the classics *Alice's Adventures in Wonderland* and "Jabberwocky," created a word that describes the kind of play Qigong people engage in. His word is "galumphing," and it represents the activity of a child's game where the rules are few, but the pretend adventures are many. This is the kind of game we all used to play one time in our life, but generally don't any more. A child is galumphing when a fallen stick becomes Excalibur and a kitchen broom turns into a fiery horse.

As children, we played so we could explore the world around us, and in the process learn about our inner selves as well. When we played as children, we were refreshed, challenged, inquisitive, carefree, and happy. Play was an integral part of our health, growth, and development. But as we grow up, the games get more serious and responsibilities become more adult. Our minds become less adventurous, and our bodies, well, they just don't work like they did when we were kids. Consequently, we stop exploring our deeper selves. It also becomes harder and harder to learn from our inner life, and when our heart speaks, we can barely hear it.

The only way to reclaim our minds, bodies, and our spirits is to learn to play again. Don't you think we could all stand to play a little every morning before we go out to meet the challenges of our day? That's precisely what the ancient creators of Qigong thought, and their wisdom was so profound that it survives actively and vitally to the present day.

What's so exciting about our Morning Cup of Qigong is that you actively engage the full force of your imagination as you play it. It's just like being a kid again! Remember: in the land of Qigong, you are only as limited as your imagination.

You are almost ready to take the first step of your Morning Cup, but before you do, I have one last — and very important — secret to tell you.

The Secret of the New Forest

One of the most important secrets of New Forest Qigong is the New Forest itself. To imagine yourself playing Qigong in a beautiful natural setting has a profoundly nourishing effect on your entire bodymind and spirit. The outdoors is, after all, where we take vacations to recharge our batteries. At the turn of the century, physicians regularly prescribed time in nature as a foundation for curing most any illness. Photographs and paintings of nature fill us with awe and inspire us because they remind us of our beginnings. Returning to the forest is a root experience for anyone human.

The Chinese creators of our art used the wonders of the natural world as the primary source of their inspiration for Qigong. I've always loved the word "inspired." It means "in spirit." As you play Qigong, you are playing in the spirit of the natural world, in fact, in the spirit of all creation. While it's always enjoyable to play your Qigong outdoors, it is not always convenient or practical. But envisioning the New Forest is something that you can do at any time no matter where you are.

Think of the New Forest as an actual place that exists in a dimension parallel to your everyday world; it's always there; it always has been. You just have to think about it for it to appear. Our Qigong forest is a lush, verdant environment teeming with life and energy. Growth and the hidden promise of growth exist all around you. Whatever you need for survival, nourishment, health, and wellness is waiting for you in the New Forest. As soon as you bring this forest into focus, all of the tools and materials you need to be at your best present themselves to you. To me, the New Forest represents a return to the Garden, a return to the field of all possibilities where you can rest comfortably in God's hands. This is the ideal place to play your Qigong.

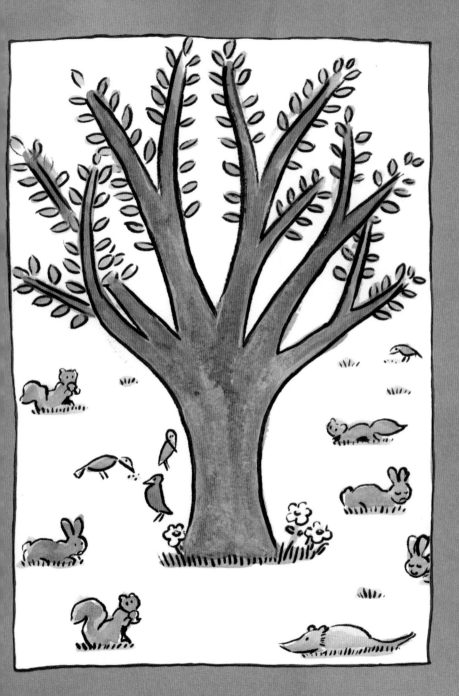

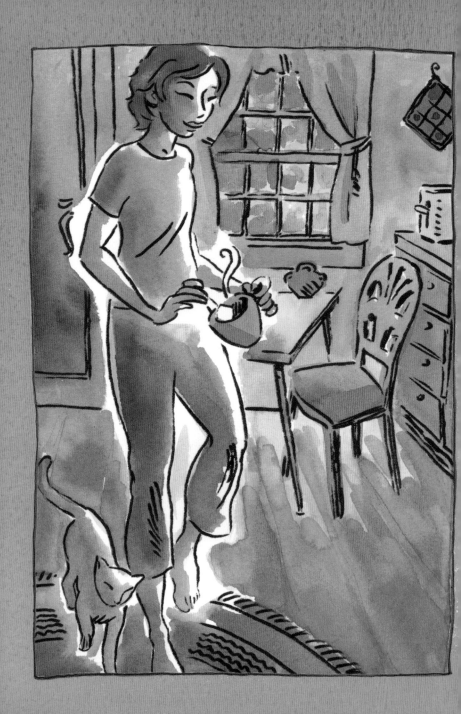

The Routine

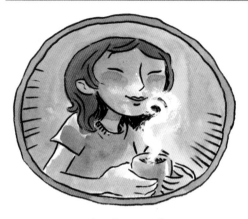

This Qigong routine can be done in about 15 minutes each morning with no special equipment. You can take more time by moving more slowly, and you can also add the extra sips included toward the back of the book. You can use the CD in the back of the book to follow along, or use it alone if you're in a hurry. Feel free to do all ten exercises, or just a few each morning.

When you opened this book, you became a member of a very elite and very ancient fraternity. As a new member, you should know that we don't call ourselves athletes, scholars, warriors, disciples, or even students. We refer to ourselves as players, gardeners, and cultivators. We do this because we use Qigong to cultivate our lives as if we were tending a beautiful garden; and isn't that how it should be? As a new Qigong player, you will begin your cultivation by learning how to master the ethereal and unseen life-force that is within each of us. Then, you will learn how to use your new skills to cope with the stresses and demands that make up the dynamics of everyday living. It's really very simple: you cultivate the life-force so you can cultivate life. Welcome to New Forest Qigong.

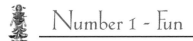

Number 1 - Fun

This exercise promotes mental and physical relaxation. Shaping your Qi with this movement clears your head when you're under stress and encourages smooth circulation of your life-force energy.

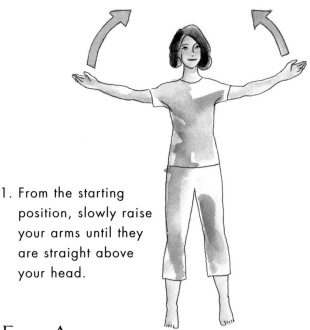

1. From the starting position, slowly raise your arms until they are straight above your head.

Extra Attention

Think about the 1-Fun internal adjustment. You may even silently repeat to yourself, "Smiling faintly, I am relaxed, alert, and aware." Qigong practitioners call mental statements of this kind "Pithy Formulas," or "Songs of the Exercise."

2. Move your arms down as if you were stroking a long white beard or gently smoothing out a cat's fur. Let your relaxed palms face you as they gently move downward, floating a few inches in front of your torso. Move slowly and deliberately without any excessive tension in your hands and fingers. Inhale as your hands and arms rise up, and exhale as they move downward.

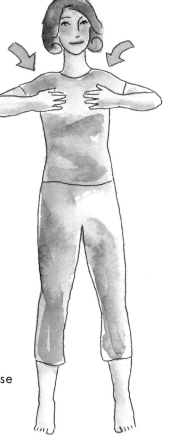

3. Play this exercise 10 times.

Extra Attention

As you smooth out your Qi, imagine that waves of relaxation descend downward through your bodymind. It's as if you are encouraging hundreds of smiles to move down through you, relaxing every part of you that they touch.

Number 2 - Shoe

This Qigong exercise increases your overall vitality for living. It also helps you preserve your ability to maintain a relaxed state as you move through your daily life.

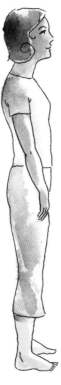

1. Stand with your arms by your side.

2. Move your weight to the balls of your feet and slowly stretch upward one to three inches, lifting your heels off the floor.

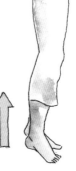

Extra Attention

Think about the 2-Shoe internal adjustment. A Pithy Formula might be "My feet melt into the earth's surface; I stand firm."

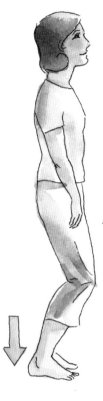

3. Lightly and gently allow your heels to drop to the floor. As your heels drop to the floor, let your body respond with a slight bouncing, springing motion. Pretend your legs and bent knees are shock absorbers.

4. Inhale as you lift your heels off the floor, and exhale as you drop them back down and let your legs absorb the vibrations.

5. Play this exercise 10 times.

Extra Attention

This Qigong exercise can readily be adapted to fit your needs. If you lose your balance, then don't lift your heels more than an inch off the floor. Better yet, steady yourself with a chair or a countertop. If you like, you can lift the whole foot off the ground and stomp it gently down. You can even play this exercise sitting in a chair.

Number 3 - Tree

Shaping your Qi with this exercise encourages life-force energy to flow smoothly into your bodymind from your environment, just as it flows through a tree. It also extracts abundant Qi from the air that you breathe, nourishing the entire bodymind.

1. Begin a gently wriggling, trembling, and shaking motion with your hands and fingers.

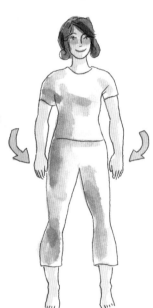

Extra Attention

Visualize the 3-Tree internal adjustment. Silently say to yourself, "I am a tree with deep roots, with wind rustling through my leaves and branches." Imagine that your roots grow deeper and stronger as the vibrations you create move into the floor or ground.

2. Move this shaking
   vibration up your arms
   into your shoulders.

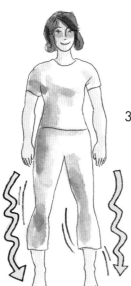

3. Shake
   downward
   from your
   shoulders to your torso, hips, legs,
   and, finally, into your feet,
   wiggling your toes at the very end.
   Pretend that the vibration continues
   to move downward into the ground
   beneath your feet.

4. Let your natural breathing support the speed of this
   exercise. Inhale and get ready to shake. Then, exhale
   and tremble from your fingertips to the floor.

5. Repeat this exercise 10 times.

Extra Attention

This shaking motion is a gentle one. Stay relaxed and try not to
flail your arms around too much.

Number 4 - Core

Shaping your Qi with this exercise collects vital body energy and strength to what Qigong Masters call the tan tien (don dee-EN), or "lower heaven." Think of this area as an organ made up of Qi that supplies the rest of your bodymind with organized and potent life-force.

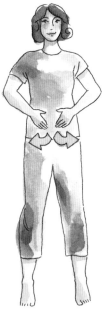

1. Place your palms slightly in front of your lower abdomen, one to four inches below your navel.

Extra Attention

Visualize the fire hydrant in the 4-Core internal adjustment. You may even silently repeat this phrase to yourself while playing this exercise: "Collecting myself confidently within, I am strong, fortified, and centered."

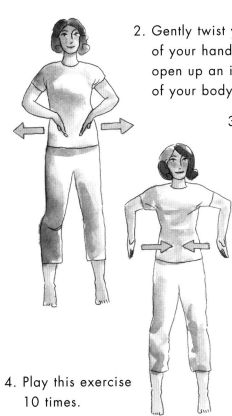

2. Gently twist your arms so the backs of your hands face each other and open up an imaginary space in front of your body.

3. Rotate your palms so that they face each other and, just as gently, close this imaginary space. Inhale while opening and exhale while closing the imaginary space. Remember to keep your breathing relaxed and unforced. Your natural breath is in charge of the speed of your Qigong exercises at all times.

4. Play this exercise 10 times.

Extra Attention

If you have a headache or are experiencing abdominal distress, move your hands up to your breastbone and shape the Qi in that position. Likewise, imagine that your 4-Core is located inside your chest just underneath your breastbone.

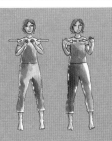

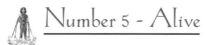

Number 5 - Alive

This Qigong exercise allows you to absorb more life-force from your environment by extending life-force to the people and places around you. In essence, you are becoming a living conduit of Qi, allowing it to flow through your bodymind.

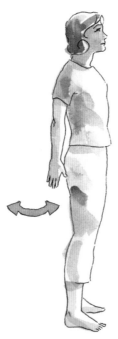

1. Gently swing your relaxed arms back and forth a few times.

Extra Attention

Reinforce the internal adjustment of 5-Alive in your mind. You may even silently repeat the following formula: "From a centered place, I reach out to touch the life around me."

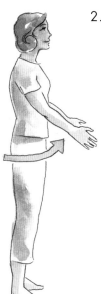

2. Reach forward, stretching your palms and fingers, as if you are extending your arms, trying to grab something just outside of your reach. Hold this stretch posture for a few moments, then lower your arms to your sides again. Inhale as your arms swing back and forth. When your inhalation is complete, exhale and reach forward. Hold the reaching posture until you finish breathing out.

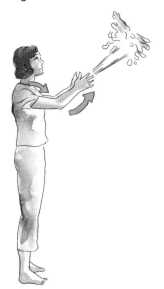

3. Imagine that water is flowing from your arms as you are reaching out.

4. Play this exercise 10 times.

Extra Attention

Keep your shoulders relaxed throughout this exercise. Likewise, your stretching reach should also be gentle.

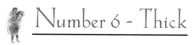 # Number 6 - Thick

This Qigong exercise intimately connects
you to your environment.

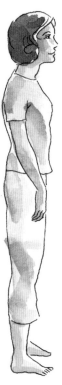

1. Stand in the basic
   Qigong posture
   with your arms
   hanging naturally
   at your sides.

2. Gently shift your body
   weight forward as if you
   are leaning into the wind.
   Let your palms face forward
   as you do this.

Extra Attention

Employ the 6-Thick internal adjustment. If you want, use the
following Qigong formula: "Thick air supports me and connects me
to my surroundings, and I feel the world all around me."

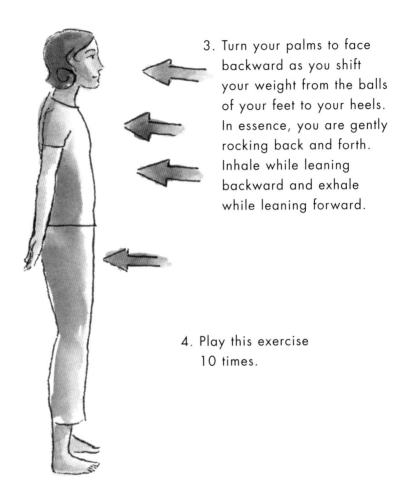

3. Turn your palms to face backward as you shift your weight from the balls of your feet to your heels. In essence, you are gently rocking back and forth. Inhale while leaning backward and exhale while leaning forward.

4. Play this exercise 10 times.

Extra Attention

Maintain your balance as you gently rock back and forth. If you lose your balance, simply make the rocking motion smaller.

Number 7 - Heaven

This Qigong exercise calms your mind and encourages mental focus by moving clear, organized Qi upward in your bodymind.

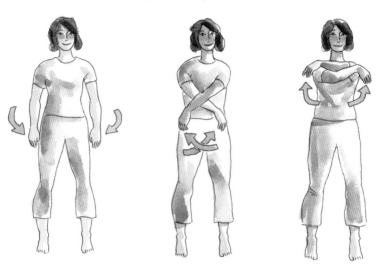

1. Beginning from a Qigong starting position, gently lift and lower your hands as shown. Try to keep your shoulders and upper body relaxed.

Extra Attention

Think about the 7-Heaven internal adjustment. Silently repeat to yourself, "A light and buoyant energy collects at my crown, lifting me upward." You can even create your own Pithy Formula or employ a short religious prayer while playing this exercise.

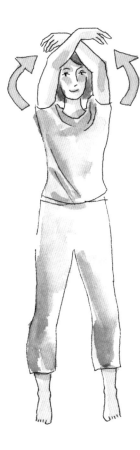

2. Inhale as your hands move inward, upward, and outward; then exhale as they slowly descend.

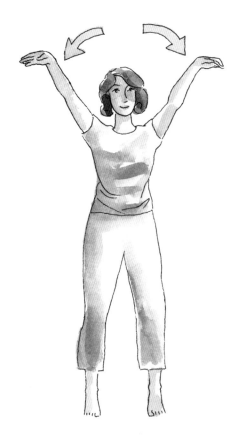

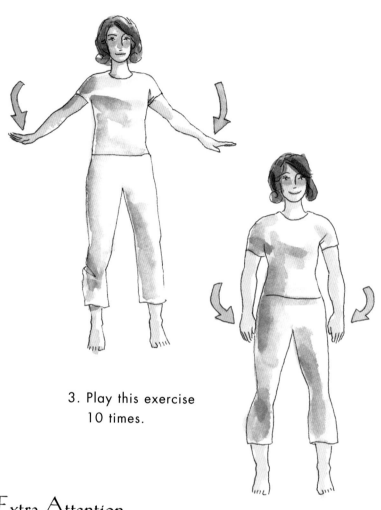

3. Play this exercise
10 times.

Extra Attention

Play this exercise with lightness and fluidity. The arms do not touch as they cross and rise upward. As they descend, allow them to float downward gently.

Number 8 - Gate

This exercise absorbs Qi from your environment and balances it out so that you will have an even amount of Qi throughout your bodymind. It also encourages balance in other areas of your life as well.

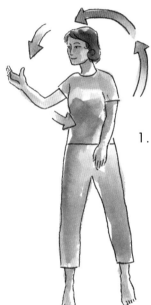

1. Bring your right hand up to trace a clockwise circle in the air. Turn your body slightly to the right as you do.

Extra Attention

Think about the 8-Gate internal adjustment as you move. If you like, use one of the Qigong formulas that follow or make one up on your own. "I gently absorb and balance the energy of everyday living." Or, "Gently, I gather the energy of life, absorbing and balancing it."

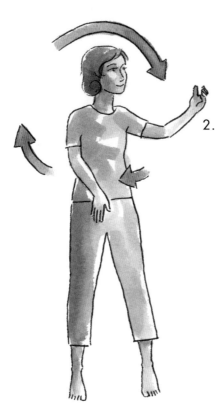

2. As soon as you have completed the right circle, turn slightly to the left and trace a counterclockwise circle with your left hand. Inhale as your arms move up their circles and exhale as they move down them. You have essentially made an infinity circle with your two hands.

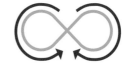

3. Play this exercise 10 times.

Extra Attention

If possible, look at your palm as it comes up the circle (6 o'clock position to the 12 o'clock position). When your hand circles downward (12 o'clock position to the 6 o'clock position), look at the back of your hand. Try to move continuously as you trace the Qigong circles from one side to the other.

Number 9 - Shine

This exercise can really brighten your day if you're feeling depressed or grumpy. It can also keep out pernicious influences from the environment and the world around you.

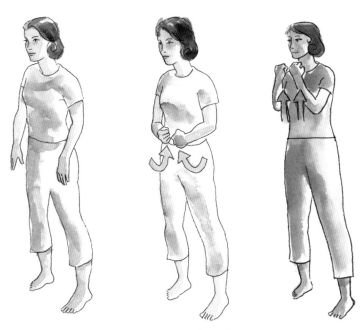

1. Bring your hands up gently as shown.

Extra Attention

Think about the 9-Shine imagery when playing this exercise. A good Qigong formula might be "Shining outward like a bright flame, I banish negativity."

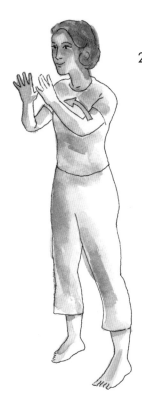

2. Open your hands and stretch your palms, arms, and fingers outward as if you are pushing something away from you.

Extra Attention

Even though you are employing a pushing motion away from your bodymind, don't use regular strength or force. Rather, stay relaxed and pretend you are pushing the world's heaviest object using no strength at all.

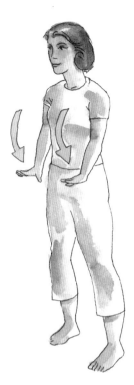

3. Inhale as the hands come up, and exhale as you press forward. Keep your breath relaxed and unforced.

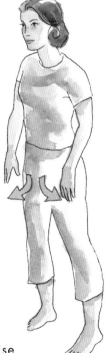

4. At the end of your press, allow your hands to lower to your sides.

5. Play this exercise 10 times.

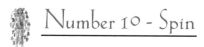

Number 10 - Spin

This exercise generates the Qi of spontaneity and creativity. It also intensifies the overall effects of your New Forest Qigong play.

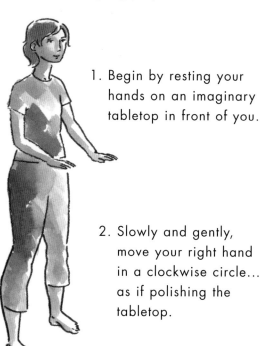

1. Begin by resting your hands on an imaginary tabletop in front of you.

2. Slowly and gently, move your right hand in a clockwise circle... as if polishing the tabletop.

Extra Attention

Let your mind float amongst all nine previous internal adjustments. Create your own Qigong formula or use this one: "Watching one hand and then the other, I let my mind wander, remembering that anything is possible in the New Forest."

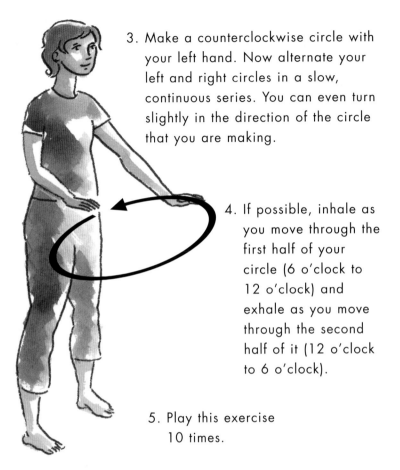

3. Make a counterclockwise circle with your left hand. Now alternate your left and right circles in a slow, continuous series. You can even turn slightly in the direction of the circle that you are making.

4. If possible, inhale as you move through the first half of your circle (6 o'clock to 12 o'clock) and exhale as you move through the second half of it (12 o'clock to 6 o'clock).

5. Play this exercise 10 times.

Extra Attention

Keep your palms facing down throughout this exercise and look intently at the back of the hand that is circling. While one hand is circling, the other one waits patiently on the imaginary tabletop until its turn to move.

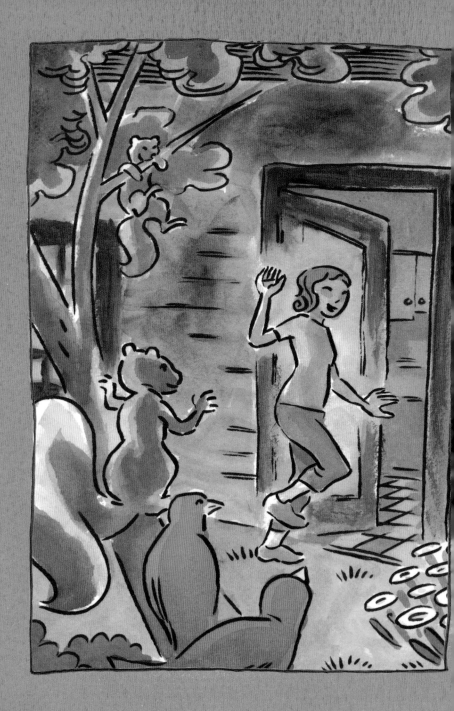

Leaving the New Forest

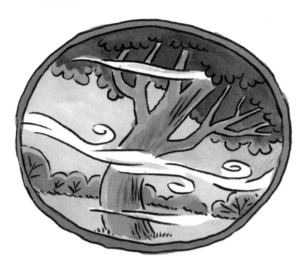

After completing your last Qigong exercise, relax your arms, letting them hang naturally to your sides with an imaginary egg under each armpit. If possible, bend your knees just enough to provide a feeling of resilience. Close your eyes if you like.

Think about the lush green New Forest and all of the internal explorations you've done and adventures you've just had. Stand quietly in this posture and review the keywords from 10 to 1: 10-Spin, 9-Shine, 8-Gate, 7-Heaven, 6-Thick, 5-Alive, 4-Core, 3-Tree, 2-Shoe, and 1-Fun.

Pretend now that you are about to leave the New Forest to go out and take on your day. In reality, the wonders of the New Forest with all the secrets and adventures will always be with you. Congratulations! You have begun to master the unseen life-force with the art of New Forest Qigong.

An Extra Sip

Intermediate Qigong Breathing

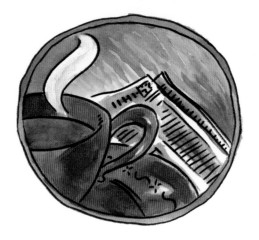

If you are interested in delving deeper into the mysteries of Qigong breathing, try the following intermediate exercise. Imagine that there is a balloon in your lower abdomen located about three to five inches below your navel and inward, hidden inside you.

As you breathe in, imagine that the inhaled air goes straight down to this balloon. As you breathe out, imagine that the balloon collapses. Did you notice that I didn't say "contracts as you exhale"? This is very important. You are pretending that the air moves into and out of your bodymind of its own accord. The air simply comes into your balloon, expanding it to about the size of a grapefruit, and then leaves the balloon, which collapses as you exhale. Further, imagine that there is a long glass tube that extends from the top of the balloon straight up through the center of your torso and neck. Visualize the opened end of the glass tube pointing upward deep inside the center of your skull. Imagine that the opened end of this tube is where your breathing actually begins. Your nostrils are merely two holes conveniently placed to allow the air you breathe to get to the top of the open glass tube inside your head.

To complete the image, see the air that moves in and out of your bodymind as finely spun silver and gold threads or filaments.

Over time, this way of Qigong breathing will change your relationship to precisely how you breathe. Your breath will naturally slow down, and your whole body will relax as your respiration becomes more efficient. Your blood will become filled with life-giving oxygen and energy. This way of breathing is one of the best-kept secrets of Chinese artists, poets, and Qigong players. Now, it's yours as well.

As you gain more facility with your Qigong exercises, you'll find that you have greater control over your bodymind. Moving very slowly and deliberately will become increasingly more comfortable. "How slow is too slow?" you may ask. My answer is, "Suit yourself!" If it takes five seconds to complete one exercise motion or thirty seconds, that's fine. Sometimes, you can find yourself moving so slowly that you can't specifically coordinate your inhales and exhales with your movements. No problem! Simply move as slowly as you like while watching the balloon, glass tube, and threads go about their business. Don't interfere, just breathe and move slowly. In the New Forest, you get to experiment and play. What's important is that you let your natural breathing be your guide.

An Extra Sip II

Qigong Energies and Shapes

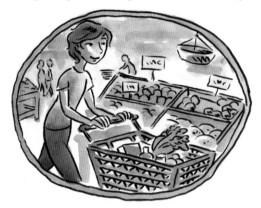

At a normal pace, your Qigong routine should take about fifteen minutes to perform. That's about a minute-and-a-half for each of the ten exercises. Of course, if you are coordinating your breath with your movements, then the speed of your breathing will determine how fast or slow you move. While it's best to play all ten of your Qigong exercises, sometimes it feels good to spend your Morning Cup time focusing on three or four exercises — or even just one. The question then is, "How do I know which exercise to choose?"

Each of the ten New Forest Qigong exercises addresses a certain type of energy that we need in order to live life to the fullest. Each exercise can mobilize and organize its specific energy when we need it the most. Advanced Qigong players even believe that they can see the shape of the ten different energies as they move in and around the bodymind.

At its simplest, knowing the name of each Qi will tell you which one could most benefit you. If you are feeling tense or uncomfortable, play exercise number 1 and generate Comforting Qi. Has the pace of life got you running around and feeling unstable? Then you need Grounding Qi, which is generated by exercise number 2.

Feeling undernourished by life? Then play the third exercise and generate Nourishing Energy. If you are feeling physically, intellectually, or emotionally weak, strengthen yourself with Qigong exercise number 4.

Practitioners of the healing arts can dramatically increase their effectiveness by playing Qigong exercise number 5 and generating abundant Outflowing Qi. From time to time, we all feel cut off from our environment and the people in it. This is an indication that we need more Connecting Qi. Play exercise number 6.

Play the seventh exercise whenever you need a clear head. Balance out the conflicts and confusions in your life with Qigong exercise number 8, and protect yourself from negative emotions with the ninth exercise, generating Protective Qi. Boost your intuition and creativity with the tenth exercise, and apply extra Qi to whatever it is that you do.

Soon you will start to intrinsically know which energy or energies need to be cultivated. Then you can design your Morning Cup routine accordingly. Eventually, you will participate in an intimate conversation with your innermost self. Silent words, Qi, feelings, and lush images will become a subtle language of nuance and profound import. In essence, you will be having a conversation with your bodymind. Once you've become skilled at New Forest Qigong, you can play a freeform arrangement of the ten exercises, guided by your intuition, higher ideals, and your innermost self.

Think about it. You enter the New Forest whenever you want or need to, take in its beauties and wonder, and then play and explore in its majesty, taking only what you need. You honor the energy of life all around you as you shape and mold it the way a sculptor shapes clay. At that glorious point, you and your life become a work of art! What could be better?

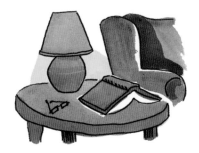

The Qigong exercises and their respective energies and shapes are:

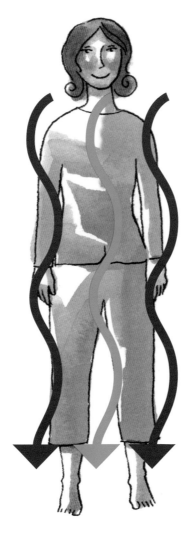

Qigong exercise number 1-Fun generates Comforting Qi.

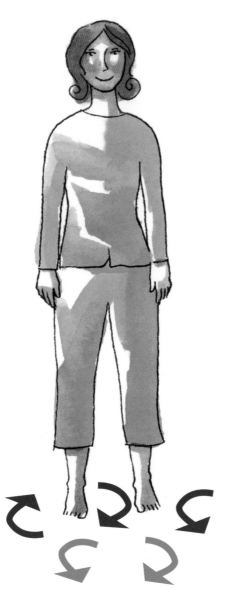

Qigong exercise number 2-Shoe generates Grounding Qi.

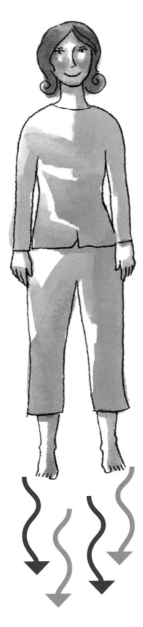

Qigong exercise number 3-Tree generates Nourishing Qi.

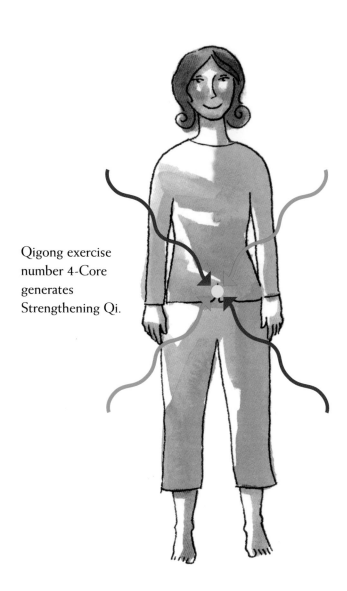

Qigong exercise number 4-Core generates Strengthening Qi.

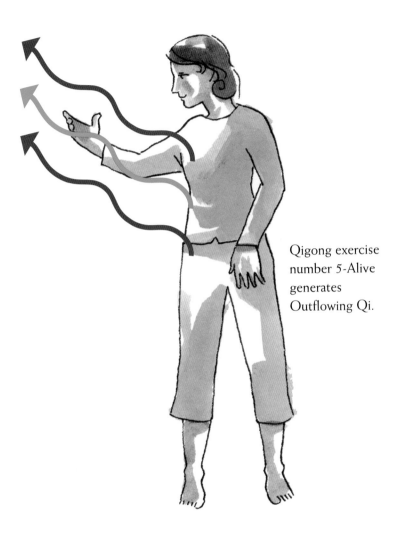

Qigong exercise
number 5-Alive
generates
Outflowing Qi.

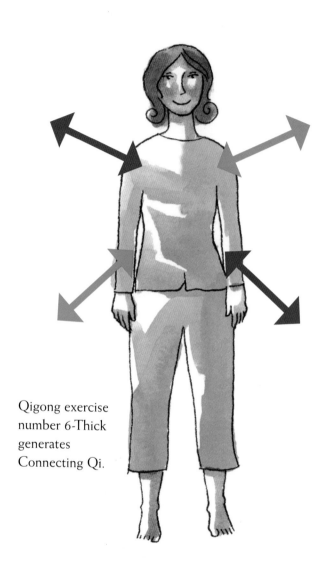

Qigong exercise
number 6-Thick
generates
Connecting Qi.

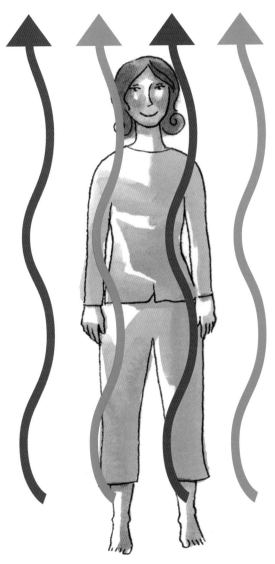

Qigong exercise number 7-Heaven generates Uplifting Qi.

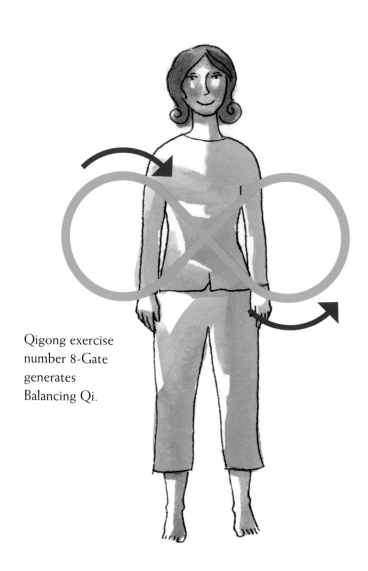

Qigong exercise
number 8-Gate
generates
Balancing Qi.

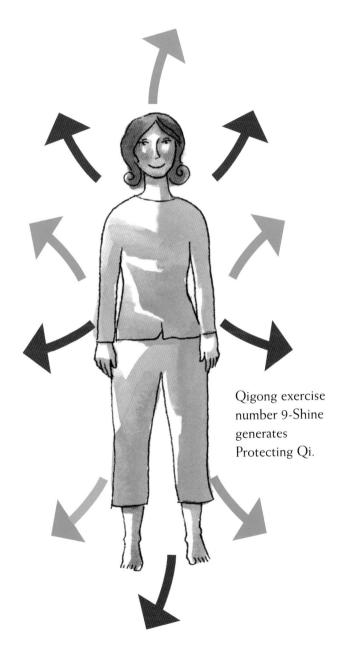

Qigong exercise number 9-Shine generates Protecting Qi.

Qigong exercise number 10-Spin generates Intuitive Qi.

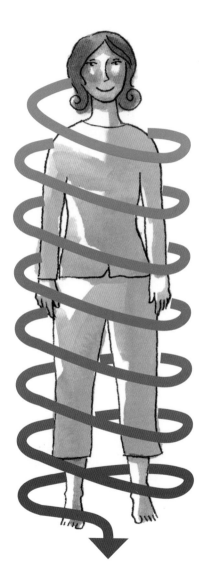

An Extra Sip III

The Aphorisms of New Forest Qigong

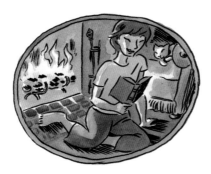

Traditionally, Qigong is a folk art passed down from a teacher to a student in a strict Master-Apprentice relationship. The student is then charged with playing and researching his or her Qigong exercise until it becomes a part of his or her life. The teacher provides guidance along the way so that the student's progress is as smooth as possible. Following tradition, I have now passed on these exercises to you. Obviously, I cannot give you the same one-to-one support that I would if we were engaged in the strict Master-Apprentice model. But I do want your progress to be as smooth as it can possibly be.

The aphorisms that follow are designed to support and accelerate your Qigong play, even to the most advanced levels. They will supercharge your Qigong, guide you along a successful path, and protect you during your explorations of the New Forest. Study and meditate on them. They represent the combined wisdom of many generations of Qigong players in my tradition. Use them to fine tune your Qigong and lead you unerringly to the many wonders of the New Forest.

APHORISM 1: Play all New Forest Qigong activities slowly and deliberately without hurry and without worry.

APHORISM 2: New Forest Qigong activities call for a gently held peak attention. Hold a quiet reverence for each posture, each movement, and each moment.

APHORISM 3: Playing New Forest Qigong is a private conversation held with yourself. Each posture and movement speaks to you directly and addresses a need that is unique to you.

APHORISM 4: New Forest Qigong activities affect the bodymind in direct proportion to the player's expectation. If you think that all you are doing is waving your hands slowly in the air, then the exercise won't affect you very much. If, however, you think you are slowly moving mountains with the turn of a wrist, then the exercise's effects become truly profound.

APHORISM 5: Play New Forest Qigong activities to meet the demands of the occasion and the setting. Allow the details of the exercise to unfold as they will. The speed and the intensity will vary widely; this doesn't matter. Simply adapt the exercise to your situation at the moment.

APHORISM 6: New Forest Qigong activities have a power, force, and life all their own. Play them with a feeling of public solitude as if each activity is so important that it supersedes anything else going on around you. To put it simply, pretend that you are in a park filled with people doing the most important thing you could possibly do, but you are alone.

APHORISM 7: Play New Forest Qigong exercises with a feeling of quiet awe at what is transpiring. You are creating small miracles with every breath, thought, and gesture. Our Qigong is the art of astonishment.

APHORISM 8: Play each New Forest Qigong activity as if it were everlasting. Access each exercise from its home in the New Forest, which is the invisible realm of the spirit. Once the exercise is complete, pretend that it gently returns to the New Forest.

APHORISM 9: Play New Forest Qigong as if it were an ephemeral activity; that is, each posture, movement, and moment is an isolated event in space and time that just spontaneously appears. It will exist from the instant of its appearance through the time that you play the exercise. Pretend that it is a totally impromptu action that you will never be able to repeat again.

APHORISM 10: Play New Forest Qigong exercises selflessly, as if you are a priest or shaman blessing all of mankind with each thought and gesture. Be effortless and empty so the blessing force of life can flow through you to others without interference. Yours is the hand that consecrates.

"The most beautiful thing we can experience is the mysterious; it is the source of all true art and science. He to whom this emotion is a stranger, who can no longer pause to wonder and stand rapt in awe, is as good as dead: his eyes are closed."

Albert Einstein, 1930

The Morning Cup™ Series

To improve your balance, try:

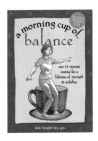 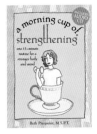 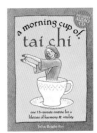 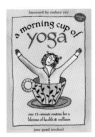

To increase your strengthening and flexibility:

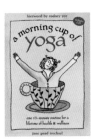 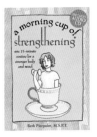 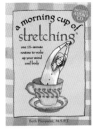 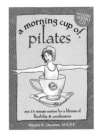

To increase your energy and well-being:

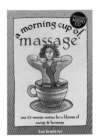 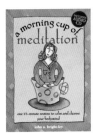 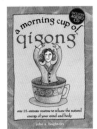 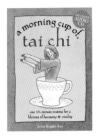

About the Author

John A. Bright-Fey *Sifu* (pronounced "see-foo"), or "Professor," is a 40 year veteran of the Chinese Health Exercise and Martial Arts. A highly accomplished Master Instructor, he practices a vast array of *Kung-Fu* styles from northern and southern China and the Tibetan highlands.

He is an expert and world-renowned authority on:

- *T'ai Chi Ch'üan* ("Grand Ultimate Style")
- *Chi-Kung* ("Life Force Yoga")
- Buddhist movement and meditation arts
- Traditional Chinese Medicine
- Taoist Alchemic Transformation
- *Pa Kua Chang* ("Eight Images Style")
- *Hsing-I Ch'üan* ("Form and Will Style")
- *Ta Cheng Ch'üan* ("Great Achievement Style")
- And hundreds of other internal/external styles too numerous to mention

John moved to Alabama from California in 1990 with his wife, Kim, a licensed physical therapist and certified Kung-Fu instructor. They have since been teaching Tai Chi, Qigong, and other Chinese disciplines to their many followers.

John's instructional video "New Forest Tai Chi for Beginners" consistently ranks among the top-selling videos in the country.

You can find out more about John and other Chinese disciplines at www.newforestway.com.

Routine at a Glance

Number 1 - Fun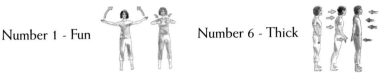

Number 6 - Thick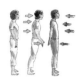

Number 2 - Shoe

Number 7 - Heaven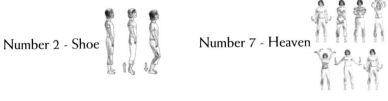

Number 3 - Tree

Number 8 - Gate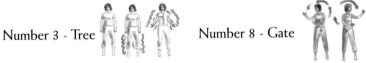

Number 4 - Core

Number 9 - Shine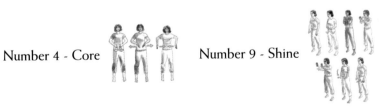

Number 5 - Alive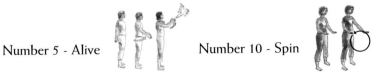

Number 10 - Spin

Tear this page out and post it on your refrigerator or another handy spot for quick reference to your Qigong routine.

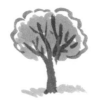